Autism:

25 Ways to Manage Sensory Disorders, Special Needs, ADHD/ADD, ASD, and Asperger's Syndrome

Table Of Contents

Introduction

I want to thank you and congratulate you for downloading **Autism:** 25 Ways to Manage Sensory Disorders, Special Needs, ADHD/ADD, ASD, and Asperger's Syndrome.

This book serves as a guide to understanding and coping with Autism, as well as Autism Spectrum Disorders. Autism is not a new disorder, but it has become more prevalent in the public consciousness in the last twenty years. Over this period of time there has been a lot of misinformation spread about the disorder. I want you to get to the truth of Autism, to understand the pathology of the disorder, and to learn strategies for dealing with Autism. I know that if you have a loved one suffering from Autism that today can be trying times, but I want you to know that there is light at the end of the tunnel. Understanding Autism and having strategies to help those suffering from the disorder will save you heartache and worry as you adjust to your new understanding of the disorder.

Here's an inescapable fact: knowing the pathology of Autism, it's prevalence, and strategies for coping will improve your life and ease your burden. We all have that key moment where we are caught up in a situation surrounding a child with sensory issues or ASD and we have no idea what to do. I want to avoid this situation from happening to you. By the end of this book you will have a toolkit for solving some of the most common problems, and will have an understanding of underlying biological causes.

If you do not develop an education on Autism then even the most simple interactions with children with sensory disorders will prove to be a real challenge. No one knows where to start when they first become accustomed to Autism. I want to jumpstart your knowledgebase and get you feeling ready and comfortable to tackle Autism and sensory disorders. Take to heart the knowledge in this book and you will have a better understanding of Autism, as well as know what to do when interacting with children and adults with special needs.

It's time for you to become confident in your dealing with Autism. Start reading and within just a few pages you will feel more comfortable in your understand and situational knowledgebase about Autism.

Chapter 1: Autism

Autism is a developmental neurological disorder that affects the brain and central nervous system. The symptoms of Autism are generally detected during early childhood and adolescence, but can go unnoticed for a number of years. Autism is not well defined and there are numerous degrees of Autism that manifest in a variety of different symptoms. The pathology, or essential mechanical cause, of Autism is not very well understood. Over the last forty years research has proven definitively that Autism is a combination of both genetic and environmental causes. With the recent discovery of epigenetics researchers are discovering that it's not necessarily the genetic code or blueprint that we are born with but how that blueprint is interpreted by our body and by our environment. Even with this information it is not well known the exact causes of Autism or how these influences exactly affect the development of the brain and central nervous system.

While the exact cause is not known, remarkable progress has been made on understanding and examining the pathology of Autism. Most of this progress has come in discovering and eliminating causes and understating how autistics are similar in their early brain formation. To have the best understanding of the disorder, imagine it this way: as the brain and nervous system are developing in a child, instructions for this essential building comes from genetic data. This genetic data serves as a blueprint for the formation of the brain and instructions must be followed exactly. Now, while we don't know the exact steps that are not followed, or are copied poorly, we do know that it is during these early stages of development that Autism takes root. Taking place around the same time during a child's development, it is the emotional and cognitive functions that of the brain that are modified during this crucial time.

Understanding what is known of the pathology, we can see that this is also the reason for the wide variety of symptoms of Autism, and how autistics can vary on a wide spectrum. There is no singular copy error in genetic data that causes Autism – it is simply a way of describing the after effects of errors in the early development of a child's brain.

Symptoms of Autism are extremely wide and varied. No two Autism cases are exactly the same due to the their pathology, and as such the symptoms are never exactly the same. Many autistics share similar symptoms, and these symptoms have been grouped together to better define relatable cases. The most prevalent symptoms surrounding autistics are language impairment, social deficiencies, and repetitive behaviors. Within these symptoms there are many different degrees of measuring severity of behavior. Other symptoms that have come to be related to Autism but are symptoms exhibited in all patients are sleep disorders, mood disorders, OCD, ADHD, generalized hyperactivity, seizures, and many more. Once again, referring back to the pathology of no singular biomechanical causes, it makes sense that Autism is so broadly defined in its symptoms.

Currently there is no medical test for the diagnosis of Autism. Typically parents are the first to notice their children exhibiting unusual behavior. They may notice that they do not respond to the calling of their name, or are organizing their toys in odd ways. They may also notice other repetitive behaviors and difficulty in the child's ability make eye contract with others. There are Autism checklists for parents - lists that allow parents to look at their child's behavior and relate it to the most common symptoms of Autism. The ultimate diagnosis and decision to label a child or adult as autistic comes down to licensed physicians. The prevalence of Autism has gone up tremendously in the last thirty years. This had led some to believe that changes in the environment have created more cases of Autism, however general consensus in the medical community does not agree. It is far more likely that Autism diagnoses have increased so rapidly because awareness of Autism has risen greatly. In the past, parents would notice unusual behavior in their children and seek advice from their general physicians – it is here where a lack of awareness of Autism among the medical community would leave the child undiagnosed, or diagnosed with a different developmental disability. As more doctors become aware of Autism, they are diagnosing more of their patients under the broad spectrum of Autism related disorders. This is the single greatest cause in the increase, but the medical community does admit that some of the great increase might have to do with a change in environment. The range of possibilities for this change is extremely broad, from pesticides used on crops, to changes in emissions in the atmosphere, and everything in-between. Specific studies on each of these causes are extremely difficult to do as research is expensive and the data is impossible to analyze without accidently including unrelated, unregistered additional causes. In addition to these difficulties, the relative impact of environmental changes is not known, however it is estimated to be very low, with most cases simply relating to an increase in awareness of Autism and Autism related disorders.

Before continuing, it must be mentioned that there has been a lot of misinformation spread about vaccinations and how they relate to Autism. It must be stressed that there is clear evidence Autism is *not* caused by vaccinations. The notion of Autism being related to vaccinations came from a single doctor that has had his medical license revoked. More information on Dr. Wakefield can be found in chapter seven, but the short version is in the late 90s a Dr. Wakefield published a paper about the relationship between Autism and vaccinations. His research garnered lots of press and the ideas of the paper spread very quickly. This paper was later discredited and the reporting of the original was found to be fraudulent. Research has continued to be done on the relationship between Autism and vaccinations and every study produced thus far has shown no correlation. If you have any fear of vaccinating your children due to concerns of Autism, please understand that the two have no relation and that early childhood vaccinations are essential to the health of your children.

Chapter 2: Strategies For Interacting With Autistics

For Parents:

Children with Autism perform best when they are kept to a consistent schedule. The anticipation of each event and knowledge of what is to come is soothing for these children, and creating and following a schedule will help them through each and every day. Set a designated time for waking up, eating meals, therapy, recreational activities, and bedtime. It can be exhausting following such a rigid schedule as a parent, but this first step should reduce difficulties you are having with your children. This schedule will soon be an ingrained part of your household, but we all know that sticking to one of these schedules indefinitely is an impossibility. As you prepare for family trips or are adjusting to get into or out of the school year, prepare for the difficulties that your child may exhibit when getting into a new schedule. This will mean an increase and tantrums and increased difficulty in social situation. Know that the increase in instances of these difficulties will subside within a few days of adjusting to a new schedule.

A second strategy that helps many parents is setting up a safe zone for your child. This is a place where your child can go and feel safe, no matter what the circumstance. The sacrosanct of this area cannot be understated, and you will want to create and define this area with your child. Try and reinforce the idea that this is a safe place for them, a place where they can go and will not be bullied or called upon, and a place they can always go when they are home. You may want to set up well-defined boundaries for this space as it sometimes helps children understand that the space is designated specifically for them. You can do this quite simply with pieces of colored tape. In very much the same vein, you will want to set up 'no go' zones for your child. Again here, tape can be a valuable asset. There are parts of everyone's home that are dangerous, but it can be especially troublesome for autistics. Use colored tape to mark these zones and try and ingrain in their head that this color means they cannot go to this area. Keep in mind that accidents do happen and that children will sometimes break rules, even accidently, so you will still want to survey your home and make sure it is safe and to make adjustments if necessary to make it more difficult for your child to inflict self-harm.

One of the most difficult aspects of Autism is looking for the non-verbal cues hiding behind your child's communication. Children with Autism use sounds, facial expressions, and gestures to signify when they are hungry, tired, or desire something. These cues can be extremely difficult to pick up on, but as a parent you will learn your child's non-verbal cues, you just have to be on the lookout for them. Understanding these cues is essential to finding the cause behind a child's tantrum. A tantrum is caused because a child wants something and is unable to get it, but tantrums for autistic children can be many times more frustrating as it is unclear what the child wants. Pay attention to non-verbal cues and finding the source of their tantrum will be much easier. Also, while tantrums can bring even the most patient of parents to their knees, remember that the root cause of these tantrums is not being understood. Have solace in that this will improve with time as you pick up on your child's non-verbal cues.

The causes behind Autism form at the same time as the central nervous system is under development. Be aware that your child may be extremely sensitive to light, touch, or other sensations. These sensitivities can cause stress, but they can also provide comfort. Try and make a note of your child's sensitivities and this will make diagnosing a tantrum or outburst much easier. It will also generally help with understanding what can be a difficult situation for your child, or give insight into what senses calm them down, whether this be smell, touch, light or others. More information on interacting with children or adults with sensory disorders can be found in chapter ten.

There are general guidelines and tips to interacting with autistics, but know that each case of Autism is very different. If you know one child with Autism, you know *one* child with Autism. The strategies here are good starting points, but remember the spectrum is broad and every individual is very different. Keeping this in mind, one of the best things that parents can do for themselves is limit their intake of Autism related news on the Internet. Autism is widely recognized now and there are no limits to the number of blogs, message boards, and forums for parents of autistic children. These can be incredible support systems, but it can also be difficult to listen to advice from other parents when your child's specifics are so different. Hearing about cases that are different from yours is not always helpful, and finding extremely specific methods of dealing with tantrums and breakdowns can often be more harm than good. The methods listed by a specific parent are for that specific child. Use general guidelines and feel assured that as you continue to engage with your child that you will create a bag of specific strategies for calming your child's uniquely caused outbursts.

For Everyday Interactions With Autistic Adults:

Perhaps you work with someone who is autistic, or displays symptoms expressed on the broad range in the Autism spectrum. There are a few helpful strategies for interacting with adult autistics. They are easy to follow and work to be sensitive to the needs of autistics. Also, if you work with someone whom you known is autistic, these are highly developed people that only have some of the symptoms of Autism.

For starters, be aware and be sensitive to communication problems, such as eye contact and difficulty in reading emotions. It can be easy to get angry at someone for not understanding, or for not addressing your concerns. You must remember that individuals on the autism spectrum have special difficulty in communication and social skills. This will translate to difficulty, or a complete inability, to read social cues and interact with the emotions of others.

If you find that an adult autistic is frequently anxious or insecure, this is not a symptom of Autism as much as it is a result of growing up exhibiting autistic behavior. Although times are rapidly changing, today's adult autistics were commonly bullied when they were younger. Many adults today exhibit a fear of bullying and find talking down to them extremely threatening. If you notice anxiousness or if they have a high level of insecurities, try and work through these differences. Be aware that yelling or getting flustered is likely to worsen a situation rather than improve it. In addition, the hypersensitive of autistics vary, but commonly touching is extremely inappropriate. We forget how frequently we bump into or touch others, both on purpose and inadvertently. Do not pat an autistic adult on the back or hug them unless you are sure that they wish to touched.

Lastly, although you need to be aware of the sensitivities of autistic adults, do not treat them any differently from how you would your other coworkers. Although they may not be able to show empathy and emotion in quite the same way, that does not mean they lack these attributes. Adults on the Autism Disorder Spectrum provided the above tips, but across the board the most frequent request is this: "Do not assume we don't have emotions and empathy." It might be very difficult for them to express these common emotions and feelings, but they are there in equal measure as they are for any other adult.

Chapter 3: Autism Spectrum Disorder

In chapter one the pathology and biomechanics of Autism were briefly discussed. What's important to remember about the development of Autism is that is happens around the same time in each child, as the brain and nervous system are developing. This gives us the root of Autism Spectrum Disorder. It is a way of describing all of the encompassing disorders that arise from errors during this important part of early childhood development. The problems that arise from individuals on the Autism spectrum vary massively, but they generally are put into archetype disorders relating to social, emotional, and hypersensitivities in the nervous system. These have been expanded and include seizures as well as ADHD and other disorders relating to early childhood development. We can think of Autism Spectrum Disorder as breaking down into two broad conditions – Pervasive Developmental Disorder and Childhood Disintegrative Disorder. The first of these is a breakdown of a child's development, or rather a child exhibiting worse symptoms over time. Childhood Disintegrative Disorder can be thought about in the opposite manner, where skills once acquired are now being lost over time.

Pervasive Developmental Disorder:

The exact classification of pervasive developmental disorder is an ongoing process, but currently it frequently encompasses four or five disorders relating to problems that start during early childhood development. These disorders are broad themselves, and sometimes Childhood Disintegrative Disorder falls under the umbrella of Pervasive Developmental Disorders. For our purposes, we will be making a key distinction between the two. I find it helpful to separate pervasive versus disintegrative disorders because they are functionally the opposite of each other. The disorders that are classified under Pervasive Developmental Disorders are:

- Pervasive Developmental Disorder Not Otherwise Specified
- Autism
- Asperger Syndrome
- Rett Syndrome

The first, describing developmental disorders not otherwise specified is the most common diagnosis of Autism, getting around half of all Autism spectrum related diagnoses. It includes some aspects of Autism, but not enough to make a full diagnosis. The second, Autism, is the most well known and is often used interchangeably with other Pervasive Developmental Disorders. The third, Asperger Syndrome, is typically characterized as a difficulty in social interaction and communication, combined with repetitive patterns of interests and behaviors – we will delve deeper into Asperger syndrome in chapter four. Lastly, Rett Syndrome is an extremely rare condition that is frequently confused for Autism or cerebral palsy. It effects mostly females and is characterized by small feet and hands, gastrointestinal disorders, and growth failure.

Childhood Disintegrative Disorder:

CDD, or Childhood disintegrative Disorder, is rare and was recently combined into the general spectrum of Autism disorders. CDD patients exhibit normal childhood development, with the acquisition of language, motor skills, and emotional skills all developing on a normal trajectory. Unfortunately, between the ages of two and ten children start to lose function of some of these basic skills. CDD is defined by a loss in at lest two of the following six areas of development:

- Self care and social skills
- Bowel and bladder control

- Ability to 'play'
- Motor skills, as well as fine motor skills
- Ability to communicate ideas using language
- Ability to understand ideas using language

It also includes the occurrence of serious problems in two or more of the following areas:

- Communication
- Repetitive behavior patterns
- Social interaction

As with other disorders on the Autism spectrum, the exact causes of CDD are unknown. From a view of practicality, CDD is similar to low functioning levels of Autism and can manifest itself within a matter of weeks or years. CDD is associated with higher instances of other conditions such as the Lipid Storage Disease, or the accidental buildup of fats in the brain and nervous system.

Diagnosis for CDD usually starts with the parents, but official diagnoses can take months, if not years. There is a lot of difficulty in detecting CDD because children frequently exhibit skills before the slow dismantling of those abilities. With a doctor's diagnosis, there are several treatment options available. The most effective of these has proven to be behavioral therapy where children relearn essential skills after they are lost. Sometimes these skills are replacements for others, such as sign language replacing verbal communication. Behavioral therapy takes years and is both a significant mental and financial burden. Complications from CDD are common and each issue is dealt with separately. Seizures have a higher instance of occurrence in CDD populations, however this is treated with medication and diagnoses occurs at a different instance than generalized CDD.

Chapter 4: Asperger Syndrome

Asperger Syndrome is a neurological development disorder on the spectrum of Autism disorders. It is considered to be relatively mild on this spectrum with patients exhibiting normal intelligence and use of language. Asperger's patients typically exhibit difficulty in social situations, with challenges coming from reading other people's emotions and expressing their own. Peoples diagnosed with Asperger Syndrome carry their symptoms for the rest of their lives. These symptoms can start appearing around the age of two, or can occur later, but typically symptoms will be showing before the age of six.

The underlying cause of Asperger Syndrome, like with all early childhood developmental disorders, is largely unknown. The exact biomechanics have been studied but little progress has been made in understanding how and why Asperger's patients exhibit similar symptom. It is thought that the greatest unity among Asperger's patients is that problems arise while still in development, and while these problems may differ, they appear around the same time a child is in the womb. Asperger's is thought to be inherited, but the underlying genetics for proving this has yet to be conclusive. Research is continuing, but even if a genetic cause is found, it will do little to further the understanding of the exact biomechanics and will not help create a potential way to avoid Asperger's from affecting unborn children.

Symptoms of Asperger's patients vary, but they have more in common with one another than other individuals that fall within the same disorders on the Autism spectrum. The symptoms in early childhood are similar to Autism, but language skills are generally far better, and while slower than their school peers, Asperger patients typically fair much better in a school setting. They are able to keep up with their peers in learning material, and largely suffer from issues relating to bullying. Asperger's symptoms carry into adulthood and social interactions are a general point of stress and anxiety for many patients. They have difficulty reading emotions, expressing their own, and can sometimes have difficulty expressing ideas. Asperger Syndrome is likely the most under diagnosed disorder on the Autism spectrum. The symptoms can be mild, and in early childhood it can be confused with all types of other learning disorders. A standout in Asperger syndrome is the common desire for order and classification of items around a patient. This manifests in children as stacking toys in a particular way, becoming a ritual that is practiced day after day. For adults this is just pervasive, but is exhibited slightly differently. Adults will follow the same routine day in and day out to extreme precision. Any deviation in this can lead to extreme discomfort.

Diagnosis typically begins at home around the ages of two to four. Like with other disorders on the Autism spectrum, Asperger syndrome is diagnosed at a higher rate now than at any time in the past. This is almost certainly a function of the increased awareness of Asperger Syndrome. Diagnosis in adults in quite common, although in earlier childhood these present day adults were labeled with other disorders. The DSM-5, or Diagnostic and Statistical Manual of Mental Disorders 5th revision, has removed Asperger syndrome as a standalone condition and it was only in 2013 that it was classified in the broad spectrum of Autism disorders.

Chapter 5: Strategies For Interacting With Asperger's Patients

There are some key concepts to understand and rules to follow to best interact with Asperger's patients. Understanding the disorder and working within the boundaries set by patients is paramount to improving your day-to-day experience with both Asperger children and adults.

The first of these strategies is to understand that *an exception is* a difficult concept. Imagine standing in line at a checkout lane at the supermarket. You are the fifth person from the register, and all of the sudden a man meets his friend further up in the line, cutting place and getting in behind their friend. This might upset you, but you understand the social context and that making a scene of this is much worse than waiting in line for an additional minute or two. Imagine that you could not hold back your annoyance of this, that it truly did bother you. This is what living with Asperger Syndrome is like – there are rules and everyone must follow them. This extends from the completely logical and valid 'no cutting in line', to broader concepts like everyone should walk at the same pace. These small details that might annoy anyone are significant issues of annoyance and misunderstandings for people with Asperger's. The idea of an exception to the rule is entirely difficult to understand, and this is why Asperger's patients are less understanding of not following protocol, or rules. Keep this in mind and pay attention for the small annoyances of rule breaking that can truly upset an Asperger's patients. Observing and identifying these triggers is the first step to avoid doing them yourself.

Second, friendships are extremely difficult to form for people with Asperger's. You'll want to remember this because frequently people assume that a friend can help with a difficult situation for an Asperger's patient, except all too frequently there isn't' a friend to help. Try to avoid making someone with Asperger's feel poorly about himself or herself by refraining from assuming that they have friends, a ride from work, were invited to an organizations party, or other social events. I have found in my own dealings that this is a useful tip. I have made several social mistakes by making an incorrect assumption about the availability of help to an adult with Asperger's. Many adult patients take care of themselves, but do not know anyone outside of their daily routines.

You should also know that people with Asperger's sometimes use unusual language forms. This manifests in simply strange sentence construction. When asked to clarify an idea, it's quite possible that the same language will come out, or a variant that is just as difficult to understand. It is sometimes very challenging to reorganize a thought using different language so try and figure out what is being said with what has been spoken. Each essential piece is there and often times it is easier for you to deconstruct what is being said than to have Asperger's patient rephrase their sentence.

Lastly, try and put yourself within the mindset of someone with Asperger's. This can be really difficult to do, but in essence you want to think about the world as being entirely dependent on logic. This means that you do not let emotions take into account on decisions, even though those emotions exist and are there. For example, the purchase of a house is dependent on many different factors, from price, to location, to amenities. An Asperger's patient will look at this decision in the absolute most logical way, seeking to get the most utility out of the purchase. They will not let their emotional attachment to a home be a deciding factor, because often this emotional attachment either does not translate, or it is much harder for it to be expressed. Every person with Asperger's is unique and your millage will vary with this last tip, but I have found it to be useful in the past when figuring out how decisions were made, or understanding the direction of a particular subject. It was particularly effective in helping me understand why certain discussions on topics that were tragic were so strange. The tragedy was not a central thought to the person I was in discussion with – they were instead much more concerned about the specific details of the event and not the human element of loss that was in the news. Use these strategies and keep in mind Asperger patients are very high functioning, and in areas where they use their talents, they can be far superior in a topic or activity. For proof of this, simply look at investment analyst Michael Burry. Although never officially diagnosed, he likely suffers from Asperger's syndrome, but he is an extremely capable individual, discovering the mortgage crisis years ahead of other investors and making a fortune through his discovery.

Chapter 6: ADHD

ADHD, or Attention Deficit Hyperactivity Disorder, is a neurodevelopmental disorder that affects a wide range of children and adults. The disorder is the most commonly diagnosed as a generalized neurodevelopmental disorder in children, and has a much higher prevalence in males versus females. The disorder is characterized as difficulty focusing on a singular topic, with constant thoughts and flutters to other ideas. Patients may also exhibit spontaneous behavior and have difficulty controlling their behavior. For many years ADHD went unnoticed or undiagnosed as behaviors exhibited by ADHD patients can typically fall within the range of acceptable child related behavior. The exact cause of ADHD is unknown, but it is thought to develop in pre-adolescence.

The symptoms of ADHD are wide and varied, but typically the disorder makes itself known around the time a child is six years of age. Diagnosis can happen much later and into adulthood, and many with ADHD are never diagnosed at all. The prevalence of the disorder is consistent across countries, however countries have different thresholds for ADHD, with some requiring extremely disruptive behavior from children to be diagnosed with the disorder. Symptoms can be very difficult for parents to detect because the symptoms are extremely broad, but these can range from difficulty in completing homework, to challenges in paying attention in a classroom setting. Most commonly ADHD is diagnosed first in children that display unruly behavior in at least two settings, including but not limited to the classroom, the home, or outside school related activities.

The most common diagnosis of ADHD in the United States starts in the classroom. There has been a concerted effort to curb unruly behavior in the classroom and part of this initiative concerns Hyperactivity Disorders such as ADHD. In some counties in the United States, testing can be conducted by the school district and reports made available to parents. It is then at this stage that parents are given options for how to combat the disorder. Diagnoses are frequently done on computers for both adults and for children. This is partially the reason that school districts are able to conduct testing, with costs being low and testing being quick. Using a computer is non-invasive and can be a useful tool for picking up on the disorder. Detractors of this concept say that the software testing is ineffective and that it diagnoses too many children with ADHD. There is also the possibility that in relying on software that other sensory disorders are going unnoticed, such as failing to notice an audio cue might be related to hearing problems instead of an attention disorder.

Treatments For Adults and Children

Treatments for ADHD differ wildly depending on the country of diagnosis. In the United States the first method of approaching ADHD in children is with behavioral therapy, and if symptoms persist, medication may later be prescribed. It is now suggested that children under the age of six do not take medication, and that medication in children has only been proven to be effective for up to fourteen months. It is not clear that after fourteen months medication becomes less effective in all patients, or some patients, but this is the cutoff in available research and other studies have shown that medications are not as effective in the long run. After the age of twelve in children, instances of prescribing medications skyrockets, with Ritalin being among the top prescribed drugs. This medication and similar medications to it function by increasing dopamine and serotonin levels in the brain. This is thought to improve messaging within synapses and aid in concentration. Detractors say that Ritalin is overprescribed and that this effect can be seen in nearly all patients, and that it is no more effective on ADHD patients as it would be on someone without ADHD. The core concept to this fight is the over diagnoses of ADHD, driven by school districts seeking to weed out behavioral problems and prescription companies urging doctors to prescribe ADHD medicines.

ADHD in adults is common, however diagnoses in late adulthood is rare. Typically other behavior and mental issues lead to the diagnoses of ADHD in adults. The first line of treatment for adults in the United States is medication, and to a lesser extent medication with a mix of behavioral therapy. The rate of ADHD in adults is not increasing, however the overall diagnoses is. There is not nearly the same community built around the over diagnoses of ADHD in adults as there are in children, but some vocal detractors do believe that medication should not be the first treatment option available to adults.

ADHD is unlike other disorders in this book in that it is the singular controversial disorder. ADHD certainly does exist and the symptoms are well known, and most of the controversy surrounds treatment for both adults and children. I have included common sentiments by detractors because these ideas are at the beginning stages of becoming a mainstream argument. I insist that doctor's orders should be followed and I've seen too many people helped by medication to argue that it shouldn't be the first treatment prescribed. That being said, there is a final argument that should be stated, ADHD in children is over diagnosed, particularly in boys, because school systems cater to the way that girls absorb information and give little room for boys to learn in the best possible environment. This argument revolves around changes in the classroom, with gym class and recess getting cut from many districts due to budget concerns and time constrains in preparing for state and federal tests. This, combined with increasing litigious school districts that firmly punish classroom outbursts is the cause of the increase in ADHD. I do not share these sentiments, but this idea is gaining enough traction that I wanted to include it for this book.

Living With ADHD

Living with ADHD does not have to be a great burden. It can be difficult at times, and patients can often get frustrated with themselves for what they see as a personal defect, but behavioral therapy and medications can make ADHD a very manageable disorder. In addition, there are strategies that have shown to help patients improve their lives.

Patients often find greater success in life when they organize their days through lists, writing down activities and tasks that must be completed. This idea of finding success through organization extends to most tips about living with ADHD. Patients of the disorder do better when they create deadlines for themselves and break down complex tasks into component parts. This type of organization is a life style change and can take many years to implement. A suggestion of many doctors and those living with ADHD is to start early. If your child suffers from ADHD, start to have them focusing on lists and breaking down their tasks. It is helpful for just about anyone to picture objectives as little pieces that need to be done individually, but this is doubly true for suffers of ADHD.

Aside from tips of organization, it's important ADHD patients have time to air their frustrations and excess energy. This can be done by scheduling a *loud time*, or time where they can just vent through loud music, or even semi-destructive physical behavior, like boxing or hitting an object repeatedly. This *loud time* is typically more helpful for children than it is for adults. Having a room in the house where a child can let out their excess energy on a punching bag or by running around is a great tool to keep your child feeling relaxed and in control of their own bodies. Lastly, suffers of ADHD must try and understand that they cannot always control their emotions. One of the most difficult parts of dealing with ADHD is the rapid changes in mood that often, although not always, accompany the disorder. Framing mood changes as unavoidable and helping both children and adults understand that these mood changes are not their fault, or the fault of others, can be extremely beneficial. It can take many moths or years to come to grips with this idea, but even early on it helps in easing the burden of these rapid mood changes.

Chapter 7: Treatments For Autism

There are many different medical treatments for Autism. The most effective treatments have proven to be behavioral and cognitive therapies, but there are also some medical procedures and prescribed diets that are quite popular for treating Autism. A prescribed diet of gluten and casein free foods is an excellent idea for treating Autism, however there are other medical practices that follow more to pseudoscience than to any true scientific measure of effectiveness. To be clear, a diet change is a great start, but be extremely careful about medical procedures in treating Autism. Some, like Chelation Therapy, are simply not effective and their origins relate back to the theory that vaccinations cause Autism, which simply isn't true.

Gluten Free/ Casein Free Diet

The science is still out on how truly effective a gluten free / casein free diet really is, but the underlying evidence suggests that it is a good way to ensure that anyone on the spectrum of Autism disorders is getting proper nutrition. One of the staples of autistic behavior is a lack of interest in a variety of food. Many autistic children wish to eat bland food instead of flavorful food. If you think about the way that Autism changes the body, this actually makes quite a bit of sense. The hyperactive nervous system makes some delicious favors overpowering, making what should be delicious taste absolutely terrible. Suddenly bland foods like white bread become inoffensive ways of bypassing the modified taste buds of an autistic child. The problem with a diet of bland food is that it is very difficult to get a proper nutrition, and the tedium of such similar meals everyday can wear down parents that just want their children to have a normal meal.

A gluten and casein free diet could be effective because removing gluten and casein reduces the instances of autistic patients not liking a food because the taste is too powerful. Knowing that only these two ingredients need to be removed opens the door to a whole host of delicious and nutritious foods. Following this diet can be hard at first, but know that unless your child has an allergy small trace elements of gluten or casein should be perfectly fine, so don't feel pressured to follow the diet exactly.

Gluten is an ingredient used in baking bread, making pasta, and many other wheat based goods. As a rule of thumb if a product has wheat it in there is a very strong chance it includes some gluten. Finding gluten free foods has never been easier as a gluten free diet has become wildly popular across the United States. Looking at your local supermarket, you should have an aisle or two dedicated to gluten free foods. This will include dry foods as well as frozen, and usually this section attempts to have the same items in other parts of the supermarket, just without gluten. The costs associated with these foods are more expensive but that markup has decreased in recent years. This again can be attributed to the increased number of people following a gluten free diet.

Avoiding casein is a bit easier than avoiding gluten. Casein comes from the Latin for 'cheese', and is a protein found in milk and other diary products. If you purchase products that have no dairy, you will be avoiding casein entirely. If a dairy allergen is a concern, note that goods that are casein free still may contain dairy. It is possible to produce casein free dairy products through a form of pasteurization that removes this protein. Good that are casein free are typically the same cost as their regular dairy counterparts.

The effectiveness of this type of dietary change has been documented by many parents, but it has yet to be formally researched. So far the consensus has been that it may help with tantrums and improve social behavior, however this is entirely based on anecdotal evidence. Also, it can't be understated that Autism Spectrum Disorder affects all individuals very differently, and a dietary change can work wonders for one person and be completely ineffective on another. Keep this in mind as you think about changing the diet of your household. There are additional reasons why parents may want to look at these types of natural diets, but that has to do more with traditional nutrition and health than with any concerns of curbing the effects of Autism. I personally suggest trying a gluten free diet and then possibly working in a casein free diet if the lack of gluten appears to be effective. It's very easy to prepare meals for one that are gluten free and the social awareness of celiac disease has made these products commonplace across supermarkets.

Chelation Therapy – An Ineffective Method Supported By Dr. Wakefield's Fraudulent Research On Autism

Chelation therapy is not an effective measure for treating Autism. The effectiveness of this treatment has been claimed by many different physicians over the years, but research conducted has shown time and again that chelation therapy is often prescribed to 'dupe' parents of autistic children into trying the treatment. The treatment is ineffective because it is based around the idea that vaccinations cause Autism, and that by sweeping the body of heavy metals Autism can be reversed.

The now discredited Dr. Wakefield was effective in promoting his ideas on vacations and Autism for a variety of reasons. For one, he sought to explain the pathology of Autism – something that no doctor had been able to do successfully, and today doctors are still struggling with the pathology, making little progress to understanding the biomechanics of Autism. Second, he used data linking the increase in rates of Autism to the increase in the use of vaccinations. This combined with a little bit of government control conspiracy, and his false ideas still ring through a subsection of the Autism community.

Dr. Wakefield's ideas about the cause of Autism were based on the idea of mercury being included in most vaccines at the time. This is certainly true, and mercury was used as a binding agent, as well as to preserve the vaccinations from bacteria and other outside exposure. The connection between heavy metals and brain damage has been well documented for many years, and Wakefield used this preconceived notion to describe a false pathology. He argued that the heavy metals in vaccines were making their way to children's brains, causing brain damage and changes to the central nervous system, and ultimately creating Autism as well as other disorders on the spectrum of Autism. The theory was convincing because it took an idea that was already well known and expanded it to explain a complex pathology that others had been trying to solve for years. In the United States and many other countries mercury was removed from vaccinations towards the late nineties, with the exception of compound vaccinations that included several different diseases in one vaccine. This was done as a preventive measure, but ironically the large scale removal of mercury from vaccinations only promoted discourse that Dr. Wakefield might be right. The logic here is that if his research was entirely false, then why remove the mercury from vaccinations at all. A lot of research has been done on vaccinations that have mercury in them as opposed to no heavy metals, and there has been no connection found between these vaccinations and a rise in Autism. All research has found that regardless of the type of vaccination, no version of any common vaccine has been shown to cause Autism – not even creating a very low possibly of Autism.

As a result of Dr. Wakefield's ideas propagating through the Autism community, several clinics have tried to capitalize on the rise of his ideas. This is where the rise of chelation therapy took hold on the Autism community. Chelation therapy rids the body of heavy metals. It is a fairly expensive procedure that is both invasive and harmful to children. Chelation therapy works by injecting a synthetic chemical into the bloodstream – this chemical then latches onto metals already present in the bloodstream, and when the chemical is taken out of the body it takes all the metals attached to it with it. The synthetic chemical is quite powerful and should never be used on pregnant women or children, and yet doctors were promoting chelation therapy for patients as young as five because of Dr. Wakefield's research. In many cases these were not malicious doctors, but doctors that believed in Wakefield's work and thought the damage from chelation therapy was worth the risk of possibly curing Autism in their patients.

As more time passes and Dr. Wakefield's legacy continues to be tainted, chelation therapy is one aspect of his research that lives on. There are still doctors in the United States and abroad that believe chelation therapy can cure Autism, or at the very least reverse some of the symptoms. Know that this is not true and that chelation therapy is both harmful to the body and ineffective at treating all disorders on the Autism spectrum.

Chapter 8: Therapy Treatments For Autism

The most effective methods for treating disorders on the Autism spectrum are behavioral and alternative therapies. These are methods of improving communication and easing the burden that a child or adult may feel when they are in public. No singular method has been proven to be entirely effective on every person that it is practiced on. Instead, each method is being carefully researched and tried by thousands of families across the globe and the United States. The following methods are not in any particular order, but of what is listed I have found Verbal Behavioral Therapy, Pivotal Response Treatment, and Applied Behavioral Analysis to be the most effective. I have had some experience with each of these methods, but it is only with these three that I mention above that I have seen real progress in patients. At the same time as someone that frequents forums for parents of autistic children, there are specific stories of success that come with each and everyone one of these methods.

NLP

NLP, or Neuro-Linguistic Programming, is a school of thought about the basic nature of human communication, thinking, and acquisition of new skills. Of all of the therapy methods listed in this section, this is the one that has proven to be the most controversial, however NLP is mostly considered in a negative light in the scope of corporate meetings and self help books. It is sometimes used to promote the idea that a complex skill can be learned in mere minutes. In practice with patients suffering from conditions on the spectrum of Autism disorders, the methodology is quite different. The theory of NLP states that individuals cannot know the true world that is around them – they can only determine what is around them through their senses and that if these senses are lying then there is no one to determine reality. This might sound like late era hippie meditative therapy, and in truth the premise is not all that different. Through the control of our sensory inputs we can control the way reality is around us and we can modify our behavior to fit more exactly with the reality that we sense.

This school of thought is used as a therapy by working to understand an autistic person's central nervous system and how they feel various sensations. Therapy sessions differ greatly depending on who is conducting the session, but the premise is usually the same. Determine how the central nervous system is responding to an environment; convince the patient that this representation of an environment is incorrect and then work backwards to adjust with the patient to alter their nervous system to get an accurate perception of reality. I have seen these sessions being led and trust me, they in practice do not look at ridiculous as they sound. The actual sessions are simply walking through with a patient to sense how they feel the world and how other people's sensations are different. I personally don't see this as an overly negative therapy – it is non-invasive, is conducted in quiet and soothing manner, and the costs of these sessions can be as low as nothing since parents often lead sessions. The lack of evidence to suggest this method works is reason for concern, but since no one individual or group is profiting tremendously from NLP, it's safe to say intentions are at least in the right place.

Verbal Behavioral Therapy

Verbal Behavioral Therapy is a well established method of treating Autism. It is well respected and has been proven quite effective at helping people on the spectrum of Autism disorders learn to communicate more clearly. The concepts behind this verbal behavioral therapy were created by B.F. Skinner, a famed behavioral scientist. The concept behind the therapy rests on the idea that language can be broken down into four component parts. Using these components it can be communicated with persons suffering from Autism that language is a necessary tool to get what one wants, or to express ideas. By showing the utility of language, and breaking it down into simple terms, children are able to learn language in a way that they understand. Verbal Behavioral Therapy is wildly practiced but is best conducted by professional therapists. While sessions can be conducted at home by parents, it is best to read some of the works of Skinner before attempting to lead sessions yourself. The ideas behind his book are fairly simple, but they are built on the assumption of the acquisition of language. If you are already able to communicate clearly it can be difficult to work backwards and fully internalize Skinner's theory on the construction of language. I have seen children that have gone through years of this therapy, and I truly believe that it is effective.

Pivotal Response Treatment

Pivotal Response Treatment (PRT) is probably the most common therapy practiced on children with Autism in the United States. It has routinely been proven to be effective, non-invasive, and a joy for children to participate in. I will say that I have never seen children as happy in therapy sessions than when they are in Pivotal Response Therapy. The basis of pivotal response comes from Applied Behavioral Analysis, and in some circles is still referred to by this older term. The practice and time requirements are largely the same, needing about twenty five hours per week each, and sessions are conducted in largely the same manner to behavioral analysis.

The key concept behind PRT is to target pivotal areas in a child's development. It is an alternative to focusing on an individual's behavior, and seeks to focus on grander ideas like motivation, response to stimuli, and initiation of social interactions. By working on these larger ideas and pivotal skills, PRT is said to improve other aspects of a child life by improving all skills and social interaction over time.

For children, sessions are a joy as they revolve largely around 'play'. Toys are key component to PRT and children will play several different games throughout a session. PRT is practiced in most major cities and a therapist should be relatively easy to find. The prevalence of the practice means that costs are fairly low in comparison to some other therapies. Note that if you plan on using PRT - you don't have to stick with the first therapist that you find. If it seems as though no progress is made after two months with a therapist, you might want to try another. PRT is very dependent on the relationship that a child forms with his or her therapist. If for any reason it seems as though a connection is just not forming, it is worth the investment to find someone else to lead sessions.

Greenspan Floor Time Approach

The Greenspan Floor Time Approach is one of the newest treatments available for Autism. It is easy to practice, does not require professional intervention, and evidence suggests that it improves mood and social interaction among autistics. If you are the parent of an autistic child or child on the Autism spectrum, there is no reason not at least try this approach.

Greenspan's approach is built around the idea of opening a channel of communication from parent to adult, and that the only way to really do this is to be on the same level as the child, and he means this quite literally. Greenspan along with his colleagues believe that being on the same level as a child makes it easier for the child to see their parent's faces. A child will more clearly be able to read emotion and communicate if they feel they are playing with their peers, and not adults that lumber over them. The approach is practiced by having parents play games with their children the floor. Kids take the lead and parents follow their particular style of play. During play parents may try and communicate with their child, and the hope is that this communication is made easier through a building of trust between parent and child. This method can be combined with other treatments and therapies and there is no cost to entry – I believe it is an approach every parent should try.

Applied Behavioral Analysis

Pivotal Response Treatment has many of the same ideas as Applied Behavioral Analysis; however ABA is an older treatment that does not focus on specific milestones for a child. The treatment method has been proven effective and is well respected. Finding a treatment center that practices ABA is quite easy, and costs are low because of its high prevalence. It is not clear to me personally that ABA is more effective than PRT, or the other way around. ABA has significantly more research under its belt than PRT, but its ideas of thinking are nearly a half century old and have not been updated. It is for these reasons that I typically defer to PRT.

The core of ABA is to improve a patient's ability to communicate by analyzing how the environment has an effect on a patient. Sessions are typically conducted using a series of props, and these props are used to instigate different moods and emotions in a patient. These moods and emotions are then reverse engineered from the patient. Often these props are used as a way for a patient to describe how they are feeling, or to express an idea. Sessions for ABA require a professional, and similar to PRT, anyone on the Autism spectrum will need to have some sort of connection to their therapist, or at a minimum not a distaste for them. The concepts behind ABA are quite intriguing, but remember PRT is essentially an updated methodology for the same practice.

Chapter 9: Therapeutic Alternatives For Treating Autism

There are many therapeutic alternatives for treating Autism. These treatments are not so much designed to improve social interaction or reduce the symptoms of Autism, but are instead conducted to improve mood and reduce discomfort in a patient. These methods can be applied to both children and adults, however their effectiveness is on an extreme per patient basis. Acupuncture could be very effective on one patient and completely ineffective on another. Keep this is mind and understand what these treatments are trying to solve: they are not a cure, only to reduce symptoms. That said, there are parents that live by their treatments for their children, stating that they have seen such dramatic improvements in mood that they would never consider not using their preferred alternative therapy. The following alternatives are not listed in any particular order, and I have found all of them to effective to different degrees. I recommend games and yoga for children, and for adults I've heard too many positive things about chiropractic services to not recommend it.

Chiropractic

Chiropractic appointments have become quite popular in the Autism Spectrum Disorder community. The reason that this treatment is effect has to do with the nerve endings in the lower back. If the central nervous system was born with a defect, then massaging the back where the central nervous system is connected could ease some of the pain of hypersensitivity. Chiropractic appointments are usually not covered by health insurance for Autism, but there are many chiropractors around the country that do not take health insurance at all, and their rates while expensive are reasonable compared to other doctors that you must pay out of pocket. A potential downside of this method is that it might cause additional pain in patients, or that the discomfort from being touched might be too much to go through with an entire session.

Acupuncture

Ancient Chinese medicine has mapped out the sensitivities of the body, and where nerve endings connect to the feet and back. These old charts are not anatomically correct, and some modern acupuncture therapies incorporate more modern ideas into their practice. There is a wide variety in the style of acupuncture on the market, and very few acupuncturists treat specifically for children or adults the spectrum of Autism disorders. According to my sources this is a leading treatment option for adults, although the effectiveness is not well documented.

The practice revolves around sticking needles through the skin to release pressure points on the body. The relation to Autism is the central nervous system and how these pressure points relate to the overall body's control. I would be weary of acupuncture as the styles of practice are different from acupuncturist to acupuncturist. If you are searching for an acupuncturist that treats Autism specifically, expect the costs to be extremely high. I would only recommend this treatment to adults or those that have live within distance to acupuncturists that treat Autism specifically.

Craniosacral Massage

Craniosacral Massages last around an hour as the specialist massages areas of the neck and skull. The purpose is to move around the spinal fluid and to relax the membranes and tissues in the spine. Again relating to the central nervous system, this method of treatment was created late in the 20th century. It is not clear how effective the method is and there are few specialists that practice this treatment. I would only consider this treatment if you are in close proximity to a specialist. The information that I have found from other adults as well as parents shows that this method might be effective at curbing outburst in behavior and relaxing an autistic patient to be at peace with their environment. There are entirely too few reports about Craniosacral massages for me to speak on the effectiveness of the treatment. The logic behind the treatment seems relatively sound, however the medical community has not been vocal on this subject yet, and when in doubt I would wait for more respected opinions before going out of your way to try this treatment.

Music

Music therapy for Autism has long been popular as it is has been praised by many parents as being an effective and cheap treatment option. Music therapy is a way of giving autistic patients another avenue to communicate. The practice rests on teaching autistic children a musical instrument and having them express themselves through this instrument. It is recommended that a music teacher that works with autistic children is used, however I've heard reports from parents that other music teachers worked quite well – they just needed to be made aware of their child's condition and be willing to work with their children. Often parents will stay in lessons with their children, helping with behavior when needed. This treatment option is cheap, takes limited time, and has a strong following among the Autism community. I recommend this for both children and adults.

Games

Broadly defined as 'Games Therapy', this treatment is simply using games and toys as an avenue to for children and adults to communicate. It is a simple premise that teachers have known about for decades – make something fun and learning becomes subliminal. In much the same way, games are a great way of gentling pushing for social interaction and often children and adults will find a game that they really latch onto. This treatment method should be tried at home by every parent since the barrier to entry is so low, but note that there are also therapists that specialize in using toys and games to work with children with Autism. If you find a specialist that works in Game Therapy, make sure that they explain precisely their methods. I have found that some therapists use this as another way of saying Applied Behavioral Analysis.

Yoga

The effectiveness of yoga on autistic patients ranges wildly. If you are a parent, you probably already have a good idea of whether or not your child could be in a yoga class with other autistic children, or if they could do a one on one session. Many children and adults on the Autism spectrum are unable to do yoga because of the complex instructions and movements requires, but for those that are able to try the method, I have heard some very positive things. The effectiveness of yoga rests in its ability to bring inner peace to patients, and this is no different with the treatment when applied to those on the Autism spectrum. There is nothing unique about yoga as it applies to Autism – it is simply a method of making oneself more comfortable with their environment; they will just need the basic coordination and discipline to be able to try the practice.

Horses

Horse therapy is not new and horses have been a tool for therapy for many disorders in the past, ranging from PTSD to depression. The hope is that a bond is formed between patient and horse, and that directions are easier to follow and understand because of the fun of the activity. It is not at all clear if horse therapy is an effective method, although I'm sure that it has been effective for some. Like with yoga, if you are a parent you probably already know if your child can handle a therapy like this. The costs of horse therapy are not as expensive as you may think, but finding a ranch that works with autistic children is difficult in most parts of the country. The effectiveness of this method has been proven to many parents and adults, but I'm not as convinced. I have read much of the literature as to why this method is considered effective and I have a hard time making a distinction between creating an emotional connection and caring for a horse versus doing the same with a dog. This might sound overly cynical, but much of the literature rests on the essential bond that humans share with horses, and this bond is well known to exist between humans and other animals. You may want to try horse therapy, but designated small sessions with a different animal may prove to be just as helpful.

Art

Art therapy is inexpensive and the consensus is that it is effective as a treatment for most on the Autism spectrum. Art therapy attempts to mitigate symptoms relating to fits and tantrums while promoting a creative outlet for patients. There are many different types of art therapy, ranging from one on one sessions with therapists to whole classes for autistic children. Success can be found on both avenues, as well as practicing art therapy at home. Therapy sessions rely on teaching the very fundamentals of drawing, and having a patient use these fundamentals to express an idea. The patient then attempts to explain this idea if they can, with the hope being that if they cannot do it at first that they will be able to do it in the future. The ideas explained through drawing do not have to be complicated – they can be as simple as a drawing of a cat, but even this simple idea can be difficult for a patient of Autism to verbally explain. Art therapy has shown to be a good alternative for self expression, and from my experience with art classes for autistic children, it is also a great way to meet other parents in the Autism community.

Chapter 10: Helping Someone With A Sensory Processing Disorder

Often sensory disorders go hand in hand with Autism. Reports indicate that up to three quarters of children born on the Autism spectrum have a sensory disorder that is either minor, or more severe. These types of disorders are so heavily correlated with Autism because both conditions relate to the central nervous system. Sensory disorders can take years to discover and treatment options are few. Currently it is difficult to get help for sensory disorders because they are not officially recognized by the medical community. They are well known to exist but it has been difficult to properly quantify and explain instances of sensory disorders. The pathology is virtually unknown, so similarly to Autism there are many treatments outside of the medical community but none of them are based on the biomechanical foundation of the disorder.

There is extreme variation in how sensory disorders affect certain individuals. There are some on the Autism spectrum that can almost never be touched, others that vomit at certain sounds, and yet others still that are unresponsive to a wide array of sensory inputs. Every case is unique and learning the boundaries of a patient's sensitivities is a number one priority when helping someone with a sensory disorder. Be aware that any number of stimuli, from sunlight, to heat, to touching could very much upset a patient, so try and find out from another person what their triggers are. If you are parent then it will take years to know the limits of your child's sensory disorder; however usually before the age of six all of them have been identified. Sensory disorders can improve with time, but in some cases they can also get worse or simply stay the same.

Children

Sensory disorders in children manifest in a variety of ways, but the symptoms start when the child is still a newborn. Newborns with this disorder exhibit extreme fits and are difficult to nurse. As they grow into toddlers this persists, with children producing tantrums and fits, and melting down at changes in their environment. To a parent, the constant crying of a child is a difficult sound to live with, and the best method for easing this behavior is to find out what the stimuli are that are causing such a negative reaction. These stimuli could be but are not limited to heat, cold, appearance of certain textures, smell, light, the feel of textures on the walls and floors, and air quality. The extreme range of possibilities means that finding the exact cause for a patient to get upset in a particular room of the house, or type of environment is almost impossible. Even when the condition is well known it can be hard to pinpoint the specific stimulus that is causing a problem, as parents cannot sense that stimulus in the same way intensity their child can. What generally happens is parents find a room, a setting, or activity that puts the child to rest and stops their tantrums. Focus on this activity to find some relief while working to identify the likely sensory inputs that are the cause of the child's distress.

Effective for treating sensory disorders are relaxing therapies. Chapter nine details these therapies, but similar to sensory disorder, there will be a great range in effectiveness across children. My suggestion is to try several of these different therapies and see what works for calming your child. For my family, it was with a mix of games and music with which we have found the most success, but even then there is a limit to what we as parents can do. Try and remember that a sensory disorder exudes into every aspect of life, including food. It took me a very long time to realize that the textures of certain foods would alert my own child, sending shivers down their spine and making them completely repulsed. I never framed this as a sensory disorder but rather just a child acting like a child, being a picky eater. Keep anecdotes like this in mind and try and variety of therapies for your child. It might take you a while, but you will find something that calms them down and makes them at ease.

Adults

Many adults go all their lives without ever being diagnosed for with a Sensory Processing Disorder. They are confused as to why they feel uncomfortable in certain situations, or why they feel unmotivated and tired. In adulthood, sensory processing disorders manifest in much the same way as they do in children. There are places, sights, and sounds that can sense the nervous system into overdrive, producing unpleasant feelings when provided with that stimulus. Typically adult sensory disorders are treated depending on the adult and their level of communication. For Asperger's patients, this means typically going into a therapy where they can express their frustrations, usually having identified their own sensory disorder triggers. Therapists work with patients to develop plans to deal with minimizing these sensors. There is no singular proven treatment, but typically sessions revolve around using this sensor to trigger a small response, slowly building each week until tolerance has improved. Some adults find this successful, but for a large majority it only improves their condition and does not resolve it.

In lower functioning adults the options for treatment are fewer. It is still suggested to see a Sensory Processing Disorder specialist for treatment options, however progress is typically slower. It is more difficult to communicate with the patient and find out what stimuli are their trouble spots. If they were diagnosed at a young age of being on the Autism spectrum then their best bet lies in their medical records, where physicians can use case history to identify their exact sensory difficulties. At this lower functioning level, therapy never proves to be truly effective. The best course of action is typically to minimize sensory inputs that are bothersome and to develop strategies for a patient's aids to follow to reduce the burden of sensory discomfort.

If you are interacting with an adult with sensory disorder, be sensitive of their triggers and feel free to ask what they are. It was mentioned earlier in the book, but again I must stress that you should never touch someone on the Autism spectrum without confirmation that it is acceptable to touch them. These are really the only two things that you can do for an adult with this disorder. All other aid will require a medical professional, and even then treatment options take months or years to show any effectiveness, if they ever show any effectiveness at all.

Conclusion

Thank you again for downloading **Autism: 25 Ways to Manage Sensory Disorders, Special Needs, ADHD/ADD, ASD, and Asperger's Syndrome.**

I hope this book was able to give you the key information you need about Autism and Autism Spectrum Disorders. You should be feeling well versed in background knowledge of the disorder, as well as other conditions related to Autism Spectrum Disorders. You have a handbook to refer to when presented a situation where you must interact with someone that is autistic, or has Asperger Syndrome. You also have a good idea of the treatment options that are available for Autism, and you know which ones are effective and which ones simply do not work.

The next step is to use the information from this book to improve your relationship with someone on the Autism spectrum. Whether your own child, a colleague, or a family friend, you now know of the available treatment options, the causes, and the ways of interacting with people that share this disorder. Feel confident in your abilities and your knowledge as you continue your relationships with your family, coworkers, and friends.

This book is just first step in taking in the large catalog of literature available on the medical history of Autism Spectrum Disorders. If any one idea was enticing to you, feel free to research that topic in more detail. I have included the central ideas here as well as useful practical information, but there is much more detail out there.

Lastly, if you are a parent of a child on the Autism spectrum, know that there is a strong community to help you – you are not alone. There are dozens of popular forums online about raising a child on the Autism spectrum, and these communities are filled with some of the most tender, knowledgeable, and understanding parents that I have ever had the pleasure of knowing. Use these online resources as they have been a great help to me and my family.

Finally, if you enjoyed this book, please take the time to share your thoughts and post a review on Amazon. It'd be greatly appreciated!

Thank you and good luck!

Description:

The resources available to parents and family of individuals on the Autism spectrum are plentiful; however there is lots of misinformation in this literature. From the debacle over whether vaccines lead to Autism, to treatments of all varieties both effective and ineffective, I want to cut through the lies of other resources and give you the simple and practical information you need.

In this book you will find the definitive knowledge you need to broaden your horizons on Autism Spectrum Disorders, and learn of the available treatment options that are accessible today. I have taken a look at over a dozen different treatment methods and can tell you which ones are effective and which ones are not. I have also provided strategies for interacting with adults and children on all levels of the Autism spectrum, providing you the key pieces of information you need to make your interactions as comfortable and soothing as possible.

It's time for someone to breakdown Autism Spectrum Disorders in a simple and easy to understand way. It's time to learn about common treatments, which ones work and which don't, and it's time to feel comfortable in any situation with regards to Autism Spectrum Disorders. Stop feeling unsure of what to do or what to say – learn the essential knowledge you need about Autism Spectrum Disorders by starting to read this book today

In This Book You Will Find:

- Laymen explanations of conditions on the spectrum of Autism disorders
- An examination of the current treatment options available to patients, for both adults and children
- Essential information for how to interact with individuals on the Autism spectrum, including Asperger's

- A review of alternative therapies available for adults and children on the Autism spectrum
- Tips for helping children and adults that suffer from a sensory processing disorder
- An expansive guide written by an experienced member in the Autism community

Made in the USA
Columbia, SC
18 October 2022

69670799R00028